EIGHT STEPS TO TAKE BEFORE ATTEMPTING TO LOSE WEIGHT

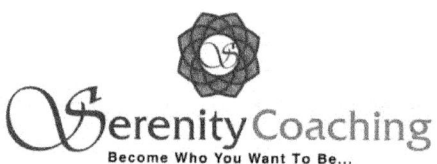

Serenity Coaching

Become Who You Want To Be...

EIGHT STEPS TO TAKE BEFORE ATTEMPTING TO LOSE WEIGHT

DITANYAN SYE

ISBN: 978-1493782888

Contents

Tables:

About the Author

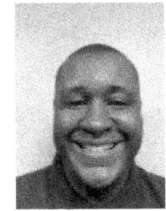 I was just like many of you who are reading this book, until I discovered something very important that I had given little thought to before—my compelling reasons for wanting to lose weight. When I really began to go beyond the surface of why I wanted to lose weight, I had a range of uncomfortable emotions go through my body that was aided by identifying what was actually preventing me from losing weight. My compelling reasons included not wanting to develop diabetes, having a healthier heart, not wanting to take medication any longer for hypertension, and feeling comfortable in my own skin. Then, I discovered that I wanted to be well and that weight loss was only a component of that. Once I established my compelling reasons, I had to face the brutal truth of why I was unable to lose weight. I had to admit that I was lazy and mentally weak when dealing with adversity. I would tend to avoid anything that I perceived as difficult. That made me feel like less of a man and that I was exuding a level of immaturity.

As I began to do some research about establishing a healthy diet as a lifestyle choice and not going on a diet, I discovered various approaches. Before, I would do what I thought would work without any research to support my actions and my good intentions did not lead to the results I desired. Journaling what I ate was my initial step and taking inventory of how I felt physically and mentally throughout the day. I established an action plan to focus on eating for 90 days and then transitioned to incorporating an exercise routine. I knew I could not do both at the same time. I settled on an eating plan that had me remove flour, added sugar, and wheat from my diet, and eating consistently around the same time each day. Planning my meals was a huge transition for me and I wanted to get that going before adding something else to focus on.

I knew I would not be able to succeed on this journey alone so I told everyone I possibly could about my desire to lose weight for added accountability. Never before had I actually told anyone that I wanted to lose weight. That way I could start and easily quit and no one would ever know. Because I had that conversation with myself, I knew I had to put something in place to get out of my own way. My highest weight was 374 pounds and my initial goal was to just weigh less than 300 pounds. I stayed focused on my diet with the occasional slip, but I made it to my initial goal. Once I reached that goal, I noticed that I seemed to flat line. So I did more research on the food I was eating. I set a new goal of 230 pounds and modified my diet. As of this writing, I currently weigh 250 pounds. This journey started in August 2011 and to date I have lost 124 pounds. Through this journey I have accomplished the following: reduced my blood pressure medication from two pills to one, learned to swim, improved my self-image, gained clearer thinking, my pants size reduced from 54 to 40, and I completed three cycling events with the latest being 35 miles. I feel better and my energy level is very high compared to when I used to feel sluggish regularly. I would encourage anyone who desires to lose a significant amount of weight to use the eight steps within this book to help you find what will work for YOU that helps you meet your goals.

As a result of going on this journey, I decided to become a certified professional, life and wellness coach in order to help others achieve their weight loss goals and live the life they truly want. This book is just one tool to help others. I have included my journal that I blogged in during my 21-day cleanse. In this journal I shared daily my weight, feelings, and struggles throughout the process. I share this with you to show that I am going through what you are going through. This journey is not easy, but putting structure in place will greatly help you reach your goals.

Introduction

Have you lost weight only to turn around and gain it back? Have you attempted several "diet" plans with minimal or no success? Have you experienced difficulty sticking with anything long enough to get the desired weight loss results? If you answered yes to any of the above, you are not alone. There are many people experiencing similar challenges. A strong reason for the lack of success may be because there was not a thoroughly planned approach before starting the weight loss plan.

Losing weight presents a tremendous challenge for thousands of people, and the weight loss industry generates billions of dollars yearly selling products and programs to people who repeatedly attempt to lose weight. A thorough pre-weight loss plan will better prepare you to meet and maintain your weight loss goals. Lao-tzu said, "A journey of a thousand miles begins with a single step." Knowing what to do BEFORE attempting to lose weight should be your initial step.

If you are overweight with health issues and really want to lose weight in a healthy way and keep it off, there are a few things you should strongly consider before selecting a change in diet and starting an exercise regimen. Many people simply choose to try the latest fad, purchase a gym membership, or simply starve themselves because they believe if they eat very little, they will lose weight. It is important to ensure you embark on a healthy weight loss journey. I believe there are eight steps you should take before attempting to lose weight:

1. Reflect
2. Collect Data/Evidence
3. Prioritize Next Steps
4. Conduct Research
5. Set Goals

6. Choose Strategies
7. Gauge Results
8. Establish Accountability Plan

By following these eight steps, you will be able to put a solid plan in place that will be safe and tailored specifically for you. This initial plan will serve as your foundation and can be modified as necessary as you begin to reach your incremental weight loss goals to maintain sustainability. Be mindful that this indeed is a journey. You did not become overweight overnight, and your weight loss will not occur overnight either. It is also recommended that you speak with a physician before beginning any weight loss program. Before continuing, be sure to download all the templates on the "Documents" page by registering at www.serenitycoach.net.

Step 1: Reflect

Before you start any weight loss plan, you should reflect and answer a few questions. These questions will help shape your focus toward understanding the next few steps. Too many people start a weight loss plan without ever giving these questions any thought; therefore, most end up not meeting their goal(s). Take some time to think about these questions, and write your answers down. Some of the questions may require you to ponder a while to really get the answer(s) that will propel you forward. Use the **Step 1: Reflect** templates to answer the questions below.

Five Key Questions to Consider:

1. What are your compelling reasons for wanting to lose weight now?
2. What questions do you have about weight loss, wellness, and nutrition?
3. What are five habits in your life that do not support who you truly are?
4. What are ten things you are tired of tolerating as a result of your weight?
5. Who or what is holding you back most?

Some of these questions hopefully caused you to really think about your reason(s) for wanting to lose weight. Identifying your compelling reason(s) is really important. Unless you are truly compelled, it will be difficult to maintain your effort to lose weight when you face adversity. You need something to anchor you in order to press through the adversity you will face on this journey.

Examples of compelling reasons include:

- I want to see my children grow up.
- I no longer want to take medication for hypertension.
- I want to take control over my diabetes.
- I'm fed up with not feeling well.
- I want to feel better about myself.

Once you answer all the questions, think about what's really motivating you to make the changes necessary for long-lasting weight loss. It's one thing to find your compelling reason(s) and another to develop a manageable plan that helps you reach your goals. The following steps will help shape your plan. As you continue on your journey, revisit these reflective questions, because as time passes, you may discover additional insight into what's really motivating you or holding you back.

Step 2: Collect Data

Now that you have found your true reasons for wanting to lose weight, you need to collect data around your current habits. You will need a pad, journal book, an iPad, or some other means to collect this information. Use the template in **Step 2: Collect Data** to help you. There are four areas to collect data from (Diet, Water Intake, Exercise, and Rest), and they will serve as the foundation for your plan.

Write down everything you eat for one week. Include the times you eat, and identify how you feel during, right after and a few hours after the meal. Also, write down how often you have to take medication, if applicable, because this is a part of your diet as well. Write down how many ounces of water you consume throughout the entire day. Also, jot down the color of your urine and whether or not there's an odor associated with it. Keep track of how often you are exercising each day. Write down how much sleep you get each night, how you feel when preparing for sleep and how you feel when you awake in the morning. Over the course of the week, pay attention to what your body is saying to you. Let's take a deeper look at the four areas for which you will be collecting data.

Diet:

Rather than go on a diet, the focus should transition to changing your diet (what and how you currently eat) to making it a lifestyle choice. Fad diet plans are short-term, and though oftentimes effective, participants usually have tremendous difficulty maintaining the commitment, because it is not a lifestyle change. It is temporary, and the weight loss results follow suit.

Most people end up gaining more weight, surpassing their initial starting point. When paying attention to foods, one of the greatest benefits is knowing the nutritional value of the food you consume and its impact on your body.

Water Intake:

Proper water intake is essential to overall good health. Dehydration is an often overlooked cause of many issues that people complain of in their lives. Most associate dehydration with thirst, but once you become thirsty, your body has already been dehydrated for awhile. Here are a few ways to see if you are dehydrated"

Examples of Dehydration

1. Dry, pasty feeling in your mouth, or dry lips
2. Dark-colored, pungent urine
3. Dry skin
4. Hard stool, constipation, or other eliminating problems
5. Low energy and weakness
6. Water retention

If you are experiencing any of the above, there is a good chance that you are dehydrated. As you think about how to increase your water consumption--and before you rush out and buy a sport pack of water from your local supermarket--keep in mind that all water is not created equal, and your water intake does not have to be just liquid.

Exercise:

The body has two circulatory systems—the cardiovascular system, which is comprised of the heart and blood vessels that circulate blood throughout the body; and the lymphatic system, which removes waste products and toxins from muscles. Daily exercise greatly increases the performance of these systems, which aids in achieving weight loss. So the question is, how do you become more active? There are many forms of exercise that do not require a gym membership, and more importantly, do not feel like a chore.

Examples:

- **Walking**
- **Jogging**
- **Swimming**
- **Biking**
- **Hiking**
- **Rebounding**
- **Dancing**

Whatever you decide to do, choose something that you enjoy or think you will enjoy. Incorporating enjoyable activities in your lifestyle will increase the frequency in which you will want to do it. I strongly suggest that you rotate through these exercises so that you do not become bored.

Rest:

The most overlooked part of losing weight and achieving overall wellness is proper rest. There are two hormones, ghrelin and leptin, that help your body control its appetite. When you do not get enough rest, levels of ghrelin—which increases hunger—rise; levels of leptin—which promotes feelings of fullness—sink. When you have proper rest, your body has time to balance these hormones. Lots of people are unaware that they are suffering from sleep deprivation. Are you experiencing any of the below symptoms?

Examples of Sleep Deprivation:

- **Increased Appetite**
- **Medical Problems**
- **Poor Decision-Making**
- **Mood Swings**
- **Poor Memory**
- **Inability to Handle Stress**
- **Inability to Concentrate**
- **Vision Problems**
- **Diminished Motor Skills**
- **Relationship Troubles**

If any or a combination of the examples above apply to you, you may be suffering from sleep deprivation which greatly impacts your ability to achieve your weight loss goals. Proper rest is essential for weight loss and overall wellness.

Over the next week, you will need to document daily what you are doing in each of the four areas (Diet, Water Intake, Exercise, and Rest); don't forget to capture your feelings as well. It is important that you keep an accurate account over the week so you can make informed decisions. Use the templates or your own sources to keep track of your actions.

Triangulation: Uses known sources of data to translate unknowns into known quantities, making visible what would otherwise be invisible to us.

As you progress through your week, take a moment to reflect on the data you have gathered about yourself. Use three items to examine your status, including time of day, your feelings, and your meals. Afterwards, think about what conclusions can be made from this information. Below is an example of triangulation.

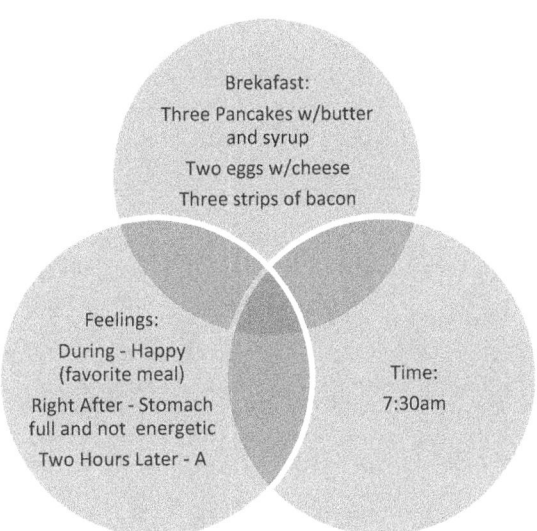

What conclusions can be made?

The meal may have contained too much sugar and carbohydrates. I felt a crash about two hours later and it took me another hour or so to feel regular.

Eight Steps to Take Before Attempting to Lose Weight

It is important to triangulate to get a better picture of how your actions are affecting you. As a result, you may gain insight about yourself that you previously never considered. Do this activity at least twice during your week of data collecting, and take note of your results. Drawing conclusions can help you decide your prioritized next steps.

Step 3: Prioritize Next Steps

Now that you have had the opportunity to reflect and collect data about yourself, it's time to prioritize the next few steps. Take some time to identify what you do well (strengths) and what you need to improve (challenges). For each listed item, identify why you feel an area is a strength or challenge, and identify which challenge(s) need to be addressed immediately. Below is an example.

Table: 3. 1 – Prioritize Next Steps Template

Behavior	Reason(s) Why
Strengths: • I walk for 30 minutes twice a week. • I eat breakfast every morning.	• Walking allows me to clear my head and exercise at the same time. • As a result of my schedule, I know I can get at least one meal in a day.
Challenges • I love to eat candy and drink soda. • I eat out too much. • I am often tired with little energy. • I don't drink as much water as I should.	• I have strong sugar cravings. • I have a hectic schedule and I don't like to cook. • I do not have a consistent sleep regimen. • I don't like the taste of water.
Prioritized Next Step(s) I need to get more sleep at night. I need to cut back on eating candy and drinking soda.	

Acknowledging what you do well can help you with repeating those behaviors. The main goal of this activity is to identify areas that are in need of improvement and then to narrow that list down to what needs to be addressed immediately. The only way this activity works is if you are completely honest with yourself. You may have only one thing to write down as a strength, and that's okay for now. Once you begin to address your prioritized next steps, they will eventually become your new found strengths. **Do not identify more than three prioritized next steps**. Your plan has to be manageable—and depending on where you are in your journey--you may need to only identify just one to get you going in the right direction.

Step 4: Conduct Research

In order to be successful on your weight loss journey, you have to educate yourself. I have provided snippets of information, but the onus is on YOU to find out as much information as possible to make safe and informed decisions BEFORE you start executing a weight loss plan. Starting with your prioritized needs, consider how much you know in order to address the matter appropriately. It is best to refer to research based and best practices aligned with your prioritized next step to help you address your immediate concern. Use the quick survey to assess your knowledge in the four areas discussed in **Step 2: Collect Data.** This will help you gauge your knowledge and the possible need for more information.

Area	Questions	Very Knowledgeable	Somewhat Knowledgeable	No Knowledge
Diet	What's the difference between alkaline and acidic foods? What are they?			
	What's the recommended ratio of alkaline to acidic foods?			
	What's the nutritional value in the foods you eat often?			

Eight Steps to Take Before Attempting to Lose Weight

Water Intake	What's the recommended water intake for your current body weight?			
	How to increase your water intake in addition to drinking water?			
Exercise	What are the recommended steps for preparing for an exercise regimen if you're overweight?			
	What's the recommended type of exercise for your current weight?			
	What's the recommended amount of exercise for your current weight?			
Rest	What's the recommended amount of rest required to aid weight loss and overall health?			
	How the quality of your mattress impacts your rest?			

Begin to think about which of these areas you want to begin with when gathering more information. Keep in mind that you cannot do it all at one time. While you are educating yourself, a general rule of thumb you should implement is decreasing your intake of fried, processed, and high sugar content foods, and increasing your intake of baked/grilled meats, fresh fruits and vegetables. Use the **Step 4: Conduct Research** template to help you decide the areas in which you want to focus on and the steps and timeframe needed. Table 4.1 provides an example.

Table: 4. 1 – Conduct Research Template

Prioritized Need(s)	What Information is Needed?	Time Specific
I need more sleep at night.	• Search internet for articles on how to clear your thoughts before going to sleep. • Purchase and READ book(s) on topic.	2 weeks starting tomorrow, June 16. Will be completed by June 30.
I need to cut back on eating candy and drinking soda.	• Search internet to find out more information on how to deal with sugar cravings. • Search internet to find sugar-free candy and beverages to sample. • Read the article I have from a health magazine on tips on identifying sugar in food.	2 weeks starting tomorrow, June 16. Will be completed by June 30.

Step 5: Set Goals

Now that you have prioritized your next steps and conducted the necessary research to gain information, it is time to set goals. Goals are something that, when you break them down and assign milestones, can be achieved easily. In this step, we are going to focus on your GOALS. When you make them SMART, they become even more within your reach. SMART stands for: Specific, Measureable, Attainable, Realistic, and Time Specific. Your SMART goals should come from your prioritized next steps.

Example of SMART goal:

My weekly sleep hours will increase from 38 hours to 49 hours within two weeks as measured by logging sleep hours conducted after waking up daily.

My daily sugar consumption via candy and soda will decrease from four servings a day to one serving a day within two weeks as measured by journaling what I eat daily.

Setting your goals will place you at the starting point on your journey. They will serve as your guide as you track your progression to meeting your milestones. Use the **Step 5: SMART Goals** templates to answer the following questions:

- Why are these goals important to you?
- Where would you like to be one year from now? (Include weight, desired size, personal activities, etc.) Do not

worry about "how" it will be achieved, just list your desires.

- Where would you like to be five years from now? (Include weight, profession, personal activities, time off, etc). Do not worry about "how" it will be achieved, just list your desires.

Make sure the goals you create meet the criteria for a SMART goal. Don't set yourself up for failure by creating goals you will not be able to meet. Let's break down the goal from our example.

My __weekly sleep hours__ (Specific) will __increase from 38 hours to 49 hours__ (Attainable and Realistic) within __two weeks__(Time Specific) as measured by __logging sleep hours conducted after waking up daily__ (Measurable).

Now let's examine a few more goals to see if they meet the criteria for SMART goals. Place a check next to all that meet the criteria of a SMART goal. Select one or more non-SMART goals and rewrite them to meet the criteria (use template).

_____ I will lose 100 pounds.

_____ The amount of self-help articles read monthly will increase from one to four by June.

_____ The amount of water consumed during the day will increase from 20 ounces to 48 ounces as measured by drinking three 16-ounce bottles daily.

_____ The amount of miles ridden on my bike will increase from 20 to 200 by the end of next week as measured by logging mileage three days a week.

_____ I will increase my exercise to three times a day.

Eight Steps to Take Before Attempting to Lose Weight

Step 6: Choose Strategies

Now that you have prioritized your next steps, conducted the necessary research, and set goals, it is time to choose strategies that will help you meet your goals. The strategies you choose should be directly related to your prioritized next steps. The research you conduct should provide you multiple strategies from which to select. Do not overwhelm yourself with attempting to implement too many strategies at one time. Narrow you selections to no more than four strategies. Use the four areas (Diet, Water Intake, Exercise, and Rest) as the big buckets for applying your strategies. Below is an example of selecting strategies.

You do not have to select a strategy in all four areas. Be sure that the strategies you do select are ones that you plan to implement immediately. You should refer back to your research as often as needed to ensure you are using the strategy as recommended. Be sure to apply the strategies as designed for the duration of your SMART goal(s) to get maximum results. Table 6.1 provides an example.

Table: 6. 1 – Choose Strategies Template

Prioritized Next Step	Strategies (Four Maximum)
• I need to get more sleep at night. • I need to cut back on eating candy and drinking soda.	**Diet** Don't eat sugar products after 6:00pm.
	Water Intake Drink water in place of soda.
	Exercise Do 20 minute circuit workout before going to bed.
	Rest Listen to meditation music while lying in bed.

Step 7: Gauging Results

You will need to track the effectiveness of the strategies you selected in order to see which are working well for you and which are not. Gauging your results will give you timely feedback so you can make changes as necessary to continue meeting your goals. Table 7.1 provides an example.

Table: 7. 1 – Gauging Results Template

If... Strategy	Then... Results	Therefore... Outcomes
If I stop eating sugar filled products by 6:00pm,	Then, I should not have a sugar rush that keeps me up late.	Therefore, I should be more relaxed at bedtime.
If I substitute drinking water instead of soda, If I substitute drinking water instead of soda,	Then, I will reduce my sugar intake.	Therefore, I should reduce the "crash" feeling I feel at different points in the day.
If I do a 20 minute workout before going to bed,	Then, I should become tired and ready to go to sleep	Therefore, I should get more quality sleep.
If I listen to meditation music while lying in bed,	Then, I will be able to relax and clear my mind before going to sleep.	Therefore, I should have a better chance at focusing on resting to get a good night's sleep.

Be sure to keep an account of how the chosen strategies are working for you. As mentioned in **Step 6: Choosing Strategies**, use the strategies as recommended so you can accurately gauge the effectiveness. I cannot stress enough how important this is if you are truly committed to reaching your goals.

Step 8: Establishing an Accountable Action Plan

You are almost ready to start your weight loss plan. The next thing you need to do is share your weight loss goals and plan with other people. The more you share, the greater the accountability. This is a journey you will not want to do in isolation. It is far too easy to stop when you are the only one who knows the plan. Share with your family, friends, and coworkers and figure out how they can assist you in meeting your goals and executing your plan. Let them know that there will be times when you will face adversity and you will need their support.

Questions to Consider:

- Who are some people that can help you with accountability?
- Have they held you accountable before?
- How successful was it?
- How will you handle adversity?
- How often will you review your action plan?

Table: 8. 1 – Accountability Action Plan Template

Goals:			
<ul><li>My weekly sleep hours will increase from 38 hours to 49 hours within two weeks as measured by logging sleep hours conducted after waking up daily.</li><li>My daily sugar consumption via candy and soda will decrease from four servings a day to one serving a day within two weeks as measured by journaling what I eat daily.</li></ul>			
Action	Time Specific	Person(s) Responsible	Gauge Results
Journal	After each meal, before bed daily, and upon waking up	Self	Proper eating will become more consistent, therefore putting me closer to my goals.
Discuss choices during the day	Monday – Friday after dinner	Self and Spouse	Provide necessary encouragement to stick with the plan, therefore helping me make better choices.
Call to see your progress for the week	Every Saturday at 10a.m.	Wendy (Best Friend)	Will have the hard conversations with me if I stray from the plan, therefore allowing me to immediately get back on track if I falter.

Be sure to celebrate your incremental accomplishments along the way. This will help you keep the momentum needed to achieve your goals. It is very important to have champions of support that will hold you accountable. It's not a matter of if you will encounter adversity, but when adversity arises, what is your plan to address it? This is where your family, friends, and coworkers become critical resources to help you in moments of weakness. Be vulnerable enough to acknowledge that you will need help on this journey, and make sure to select the right people to support you. You should not select people who will put you down and make you feel bad about yourself. You want people who will have those difficult conversations with you as needed but will deliver them in a loving and supportive way.

Eight Steps to Take Before Attempting to Lose Weight

Conclusion

Now it's time to put it all together and begin your journey. Let's recap what you have done thus far. You have reflected on your current situation to find your compelling reasons for wanting to lose weight, collected data on your habits, triangulated your data to gain additional insight, prioritized what needs to be addressed immediately, conducted the necessary research, set SMART goals, selected strategies, identified how results will be gauged, and developed your accountability action plan. By now, you should feel empowered to take the necessary steps that will work for you to help with your weight loss goals. As you continue to meet these goals, start the process again on other areas that need improvement. You will find it easier to identify where you need to address next based on the results you have achieved.

I cannot stress enough how important it is to educate yourself. The more you know, the better decisions you will make to achieve continued success on your journey. The four areas (Diet, Water Intake, Exercise, and Rest) are the essential components of any healthy weight loss plan and critical for overall wellness. You will have to decide what will work best for you. It may be too much to focus on your diet and do continuous exercises at the same time. Acquiring a taste for water may be a significant challenge for you and you have to find strategies that will promote an increase in your daily water intake. You may not be able to afford a new mattress right now, but ask yourself if you are doing other things to assist in getting proper rest. Keep in mind that this is a journey, and everything that needs to be addressed in the four areas will happen over time if you stay focused. Once you accomplish a goal, repeat the process to achieve new goals. I wish you well on your journey, and implore you to use all the tools available to you to meet your goals. Take your first step NOW!

Resources:

Templates and Coaching Services

www.serenitycoach.net - Create an account by registering to access all the templates mentioned in the book. In addition to the templates, you will have access to additional resources to assist you on your journey. If you are interested in receiving more support such as Professional, Life and/or Wellness coaching, register online or call to set up your free phone consultation.

Diet Consideration:

Meal	Protien		Vegetables /Dairy	Starchy Vegetable, Grain, Fruit	Time Specific
Break-fast	Male 6oz	Female 4oz	2oz of dairy or substitute for 2 additional oz of protien	1 cup of grain or ½ cup of starchy vegetable 1 medium sized fruit	
Lunch	Male 6oz	Female 4oz	1 cup of cooked 1 cup of raw	Choose 1: 1 cup of grain, ½ cup starchy vegetable, or fruit	4 hours after break-fast
Dinner	Male 6oz	Female 4oz	1 cup of cooked 1 cup of raw	Choose 1: 1 cup of grain or ½ cup starchy vegetable	5 hours after lunch

*All foods are prepared without flour or added sugarcane and artificial sweeteners. Resource:

http://www.foodaddictsanonymous.org/faa-food-plan

Water Intake Considerations:

Amount	Time Specific	Resource
16 ounces	Upon waking	http://amazingwellnessmag.com/7-hidden-causes-of-weight-gain/
Sip periodically	1 hour after breakfast	
16 ounces	1 hour before Lunch	
Sip periodically	1 hour after	
16 ounces	1 hour before dinner	
Sip periodically	1 hour after	
8 ounces	Before bedtime	

Exercise Considerations:

Activity	Time Specific	Resource
Walking	30 – 60 minutes	http://www.sharecare.com/health/walking/article/walking-benefits
Rebounding	10 – 15 minutes	http://rebound-air.com/best_rebounding_33_ways.htm
Swimming	30 minutes	http://health.howstuffworks.com/wellness/aging/retirement/10-health-benefits-of-swimming.htm
Cycling	30 – 60 minutes	http://news.discovery.com/adventure/the-top-7-health benefits-of-cycling.htm

Consult with your doctor before attempting any exercise regimen.

Rest Considerations:

Action	Time Specific	Resource
Assess the quality of your mattress	As soon as possible	http://www.huffingtonpost.com /dr-robert-oexman/mattresses-sleep_b_1951930.html
Quality Sleep	6 – 8 hours of uninterrupted sleep	http://psychcentral.com/lib/20 11/12-ways-to-shut-off-your-brain-before-bedtime/
Turn TV off	1 hour before bedtime	https://www.stronginstitute.com /resources/sleep-hygiene-tips-for-the-rei-sleep-program/habits-that-support-optimal-sleep.html
Meditation	Right before bedtime	http://www.huffingtonpost.com /2010/08/12/better-sleep-through-medi_n_676353.html

Appendix

21 Day Cleanse for Continued Weight Loss and Awareness

Back in February 2013, I came across an article in *Amazing Wellness* entitled "7 Causes of Weight Gain" http://amazingwellnessmag.com/7-hidden-causes-of-weight-gain/. Up to that point, I was already on my weight loss journey, had lost about 84 pounds, and my weight was 290 pounds. I noticed my weight loss was becoming stagnant even though I was maintaining my no flour, no sugar eating plan and staying active via cycling, exercising, and martial arts. When I came across the article, I was ready for new information to help me continue my journey. The article called for removing seven foods from my diet that could cause weight gain or prevent weight loss for three weeks. After the three weeks—and maintaining a consistent water intake regimen—I reintroduced the foods one at a time to see if my body had an intolerance. At the end of three weeks, I weighed 273 pounds, having lost another 17 pounds. Those were not three easy weeks. I had my temptations along the way, but I made it through.

I noticed I felt better and did reintroduce some of the food back into my diet but have eliminated some for good. At the end of the three weeks, I said I would cleanse at least three times a year and start again in June. My regimen will be a shake and fruit for breakfast, a meal for lunch, a shake and fruit for dinner, and a snack as needed. I will share my daily weight, what I ate, and my feelings throughout the day. Maybe my 21 day cleanse journal will inspire someone to take the necessary steps to begin their journey.

Eight Steps to Take Before Attempting to Lose Weight

Day 1

My current weight is 268 pounds. I had my Vega One shake with an orange at about 8 a.m. and bounced on my rebounder for 10 minutes. I packed my lunch (baked chicken thighs, kale, brown rice, and raw carrots) just in case I left before I ate. Around 11 a.m., I felt a little hungry and had an apple as a snack. I was not consuming my water as I should have after breakfast, as mentioned in the article. I had lunch in the house around 12:30 p.m. I felt fulfilled but not stuffed and was ready to head out to enjoy my Saturday. I made sure I had my shake and fruit packed in my bag for dinner as well as plenty of water in my vehicle to hold me through the day.

I met up with a friend and we were in the heat playing miniature golf at around 1:30 p.m., and I was consuming my water at the pace I should. I continued to drink water as we left to go bowling at around 3:00 p.m. While in the bowling alley, my friend decided to have some nachos. I instantly felt an urge to indulge, but I just took my attention off of them and focused on the game and drinking my water. I accompanied my friend to dinner around 6:00 p.m. and helped her make a better decision on her dinner selection. As she ate, I consumed my apple, a handful of almonds, and my shake. I continued to drink my water after dinner and did not have a hunger sensation the rest of the evening.

Day 2

I weighed in today at 266 pounds. I woke up feeling pretty good and drank 16 ounces of water as soon as I got out of bed. I had my protein shake with an apple at about 8:30 a.m. I decided I would ride my bike today for about an hour to burn a few additional calories. Before leaving, I packed my lunch (8 ounces of baked chicken thighs, one cup of brown rice, and two cups of raw carrots) just in case I wouldn't make it home before it was time for me to eat again. My hour ride turned into three hours, and I ate my lunch while I was out riding. I ended up riding just over 18 miles and burned 1668 calories.

If you want to see the results, check out my FB page at:

https://www.facebook.com/SerenityCoachingLLC?ref=hl

I was able to consume plenty of water today as I was riding. When I returned home around 3:00 p.m., I had a snack using my Yonanas machine to turn frozen fruit (frozen bananas and pineapples) into an ice cream-like treat. Yummy!!! I started doing some work and slacked up on my water consumption up until I had my shake, apple, and handful of almonds for dinner at around 6:00 p.m. My energy level was still pretty high, so I decided I would bounce on my rebounder for 10 minutes. I picked up my water consumption and had 4 ounces of water prior to going to bed.

Day 3

I weighed in at 266 pounds today. I woke up feeling well rested and drank 16 ounces of water upon getting out of bed. Today was a work day and I am usually able to stay consistent with my water intake and eating throughout the day. I had my shake and apple at 8:00 a.m. and started drinking my water about an hour afterwards. My energy level was good. Around 11:00, I became hungry, and I drank 16 ounces of water and the feeling was suppressed. I had lunch (eight ounces of baked chicken, one cup of broccoli, one cup of raw carrots, and one cup of brown rice) at noon in the cafeteria at work and had an urge to eat some potato chips. While I was eating my healthy lunch, I was still thinking about those chips. That's probably why when I finished eating, I still felt hungry. I didn't get the chips, but they were still on my mind. About an hour later, I still was feeling the hunger sensation, so I decided that it would be a perfect time to eat my apple as a snack. The apple ended my hunger sensation, and I continued to drink my water. I typically don't eat after 6:00p.m., so I had my final shake with almonds and an apple at 5:30 p.m. My energy was still pretty good, and I went to my martial arts class to get in a good workout. After the workout, I didn't have another hunger sensation and continued to consume water. I ended the night by drinking four ounces of water right before bedtime.

Day 4

Today's weigh in was 265 pounds. I woke up before the alarm today and felt well rested. I drank 10 ounces of water when I got out of bed, because I forgot to fill my cup before going to bed. I had my shake and an apple around 8:00 a.m. At 9:00, I started drinking my water up until lunch. I forgot to mention in the previous days that I only drink distilled water throughout the day and coconut water with my shakes. I was able to make it to lunch without feeling hungry. My lunch was the same as yesterday (eight ounces of baked chicken, one cup of broccoli, one cup of raw carrots, and one cup of brown rice). My energy level was good throughout the day, and I had an apple as a snack around 3:00 p.m. I had a late meeting at work but was still able to have my shake, almonds, and apple by 6:00 p.m. I made it through the workday without having a hunger sensation between meals. While watching TV at home, the numerous food commercials did spark a sensation. I just continued to drink my water and really not focus on the commercials. Before going to bed, I had four ounces of water. Aside from the commercials, I had a really good day.

Day 5

Today's weigh in was 265 pounds. I'm not looking to lose a pound a day. Healthy weight loss is between 1-3 pounds a week. I have been active, so it may accelerate the shedding of pounds this week. I have been able to stick to the routine so far and the hunger sensations are becoming less and less. I checked my blood pressure this morning, and it was 117/83. That is a great number, since I currently take one pill (it used to be two) to help keep it in check. I woke up feeling refreshed and had my 16 ounces of water when I got out of bed. Then I bounced on my rebounder for 12 minutes. My eating times are pretty much the same each day. I had the first shake at 8:00 a.m. with an apple, lunch (baked chicken, brown rice, broccoli, and raw carrots) at noon, and my dinner shake and apple at 6:00 p.m. My water consumption was good throughout the day. I have noticed since Day 2 that my urine is clear and also I have experienced an ease of bowel movements. Hope that wasn't TMI, but a proper diet should be an ease to the body. I went to my martial arts class today, had a good workout, and consumed plenty of water there. I had my final four ounces of water before bed. I've noticed that I have been able to drift off to sleep faster since starting this process.

Day 6

Today's weigh in was 262 lbs. I was so eager to get on the scale this morning because of the good workout from the night before. I forgot to drink my water and take my blood pressure pill when I got out of bed. I stepped on the scale 3 different times just to be sure it was accurate. This is the lowest weight I have ever been since starting my weight loss journey. This serves as extra motivation to make it through the remaining 15 days. At 8:00 a.m., I gladly had my shake and apple this morning and they each taste a little bit sweeter today. I drank 32 ounces of water between 9:00 and 11:00 a.m. At noon, I had the same thing for lunch that I had the previous two days. My routine for eating and drinking has been very consistent thus far. There is more structure to my day during the work week, which makes it easier to stay consistent. As a snack, I had a serving size of raw almonds at 2:30p.m. My energy level was good since I woke up and lasted throughout the day. I continued to drink my water, had my shake, and apple for dinner at 5:30p.m. At around 6:30 p.m., I started drinking water again and continued until I went to bed around 10:00p.m.

Day 7

Today's weigh in was 264 lbs. It must have been water weight I lost yesterday. Weight can fluctuate at times, so I am not concerned. I did take my medicine and drank 16 ounces of water this morning. In addition to bouncing on my rebounder, I added in a push-up routine using the Perfect Push-up. My energy level was great, and I had my shake and an apple around 8:00 a.m. I consistently drank my water throughout the day and had my lunch at noon. For a snack, I had some almonds and had my shake and apple for dinner. I am making it through the day pretty well now without having hunger sensations between meals. When I went home, I did two sets of the Perfect Push-up, and I really feel it. Whew! I continued to drink my water and made sure I had four ounces right before bed.

Day 8

Today's weigh in was 261 lbs. Today makes it one week since I started cleansing, and I have lost 7 lbs. I am really happy about the progress I have made and the ability to focus thus far with the level of consistency. A few weeks prior to starting, I was having some difficulties staying consistent with my eating plan. I feel a renewed level of commitment since I made it through the week without a setback. Since completely removing the 7 foods again, I feel energized with a greater sense of awareness. This morning, I had my 16 ounces of water and the shake, but I ran out of apples. I did two sets of the Perfect Push-up and really feel it in my chest. I consistently drank my water up until lunch. Today I had salmon, broccoli, raw carrots, and brown rice. For a snack, I had almonds. I had my shake and an apple (went to the market) for dinner. My energy level was good throughout day. I continued to drink my water up to my bedtime and had four ounces of water just before going to sleep. I am turning in earlier tonight to get well rested for my 36-mile cycling event tomorrow.

Day 9

Today's weigh in was the same as yesterday—261 lbs. I woke up feeling well rested and drank 16 ounces of water with my blood pressure medicine. Today was my 35-mile cycling event. Before leaving the house, I did one set of the Perfect Push-up. I was still feeling sore from the reps from the previous days, so I just did the one set. I had my shake a little earlier today with a banana because the cycling event started at 8:00 a.m. During the bike ride, I consumed plenty of water. Today's eating was slightly different as a result of the intense workout from riding. I had four bananas between 8:00 a.m. and noon for replenishment. I packed my lunch (salmon, broccoli, brown rice, and raw carrots) and a shake to give myself options at lunch time.

I finished the event at noon and made the mistake of eating my lunch instead of drinking the shake. The event allowed me to burn over 3000 calories, and after that type of workout, a dense meal like that was not appropriate. I was not able to eat it all. After the event, I did not immediately start drinking water again, and I ended up getting a very painful cramp in my right leg while I was out and about. I went to the market and purchased two bananas, and after I ate them, I did not cramp up anymore. My water intake picked up after I ate the bananas. I had my shake for dinner at 5:30 p.m. Since I consumed so many bananas today, I decided I didn't need an additional piece of fruit with my shake. I continued to drink my water until I went to bed and four ounces before I went to sleep.

Day 10

Today's weigh in was 258 lbs. Burning over 3,000 calories helped me lose 3 lbs. I woke up feeling good and really excited to see that I am down 10 lbs. since I started. I drank 16 ounces of water with my medication when I got out of bed. I did one set of the Perfect Push-up before having my shake and apple for breakfast. The push-ups are getting a little easier to do. At noon, I had lunch (salmon, kale, brown rice, and raw carrots). I did not do a good job today of drinking my water while at work. By the time 3:00 p.m. came, I noticed I only consumed 20 ounces. I normally would have consumed at least 48 ounces by the same time at work. For a snack, I had some raw almonds. When I went home, I did another set of the Perfect Push-up before having my shake and apple for dinner. I went to my martial arts class and had a light workout. I started drinking more water up to bedtime and had four ounces before I went to sleep. My energy level was great throughout the day. I will do a better job with the water tomorrow.

Day 11

Today's weigh in was 258 lbs. I slept well and felt well rested. Drinking 16 ounces upon getting out of bed every day is not always easy, but I did it. Some days, it's just not easy to consume that much water at one time. I did one set (8, 6, and 4 reps within 2 minutes) of the Perfect Push-up and bounced on my rebounder for 10 minutes. I'm doing the push-ups to gain some definition in my upper body as I shed weight. I have never done push-ups on a regular basis, but I know it's one of the best exercises to develop your upper body. For breakfast, I had my shake and an apple. My water intake was back on schedule today at work. I drank 56 ounces throughout the day. For lunch, I had my world famous turkey burger with brown rice, kale, and raw carrots. While at work, I saw two of my colleagues at different points in the day eating a bag of potato chips. It sent an urge in me that I dealt with for a few hours before my mind was completely off eating chips. I reminded myself of what I have accomplished so far and that I was now only 28 lbs. away from my goal. Almonds were on the menu today for my snack, which helped transition my thinking away from the chips. For dinner, I had my shake and apple. I did a second set of the Perfect Push-up and could not complete the third. I continued to drink water up to bedtime and had four ounces before going to sleep.

Day 12

Today's weigh in was 257 lbs. I woke up before the alarm went off this morning and felt full of energy. I drank 16 ounces of water with my medication when I got out of bed. My blood pressure read 118/69 today. That is drastically better than how it read about a year ago with readings around 160/110. I did one set of the Perfect Push-up and bounced on my rebounder for 10 minutes. I am now a few days into my second week. During the second and third weeks of cleansing, I can switch to two meals and one shake or stay with the two shakes and one meal. I prefer to do the two shakes and a meal for the duration of the cleanse. I had my shake and apple for breakfast. My water intake was good throughout the day. For lunch, I had turkey burgers, brown rice, kale, and raw carrots. After lunch, I went on a 20-minute walk with a coworker. I had a little hiccup for dinner. The apple I ate for breakfast was actually the one I packed for dinner. I left my morning apple in the house. I met up with a friend to check out a movie after work and I had a little difficulty finding a store that sold fruit. I was able to come across a 7-Eleven and purchased a banana. This is why planning is so important. I also read the article again I shared in Day 1 and apparently I misread the amount of water to consume before bed. I have been drinking four ounces and it should have been eight. I made the correction this evening. I did a second set of the Perfect Push-up and had my eight ounces of water before going to sleep.

Day 13

Today's weigh in was 257. I woke up feeling well rested today and drank 16 ounces of water with my medication when I got out of bed. I had my shake and apple for breakfast. Today I didn't do my morning exercise, because I had to cook my food for lunch today. I had a series of meetings today at work, and my water consumption was not consistent. I drank about 20 ounces before lunch and very little afterwards. As a result of the meetings, I had lunch an hour later than usual. Toward the end of the workday, I began not feeling well. I had a slight headache, a spasm in my face, and felt lightheaded. I still felt weird when I got off work and as a precautionary measure, I went to Patient First. Within my family, there is a history of strokes and my brother is currently in the hospital recovering from a stroke. I did not want to take this lightly. The doctor made me do several tasks to check for signs of a stroke, and I didn't show any signs. My blood tests and EKG were both normal. I was advised to take some Tylenol for my headache. I drank my shake when I returned home and decided not to do any exercise this evening. I continued to drink water up until bedtime and had eight ounces before going to bed.

Day 14

Today's weigh in was 258 lbs. I woke up this morning feeling much better than yesterday and I felt well rested. Today I decided to start my chi gung breathing exercises again since I noticed feeling some tension in my neck and shoulder area. I haven't done them for about two weeks. The exercises help relieve tension within the body and help with relaxation as well. My body definitely informed me of how I had regressed, because it was a struggle to get through the exercises with good form. I also bounced on my rebounder for 10 minutes and did a set of the Perfect Push-up. The entire exercise routine took about 30 minutes to complete. For breakfast, I had my shake and an apple. I wasn't able to drink as much today because I had to conduct a full day workshop. For lunch, I had a burrito bowl from Chipotle with chicken, brown rice, lettuce and tomatoes. That was just a little different from what I have been eating since Day 1. I really felt like myself again yesterday, and my energy level was good throughout the day. I had to buy some new jeans today, because I cannot get away with wearing the pair I had on again. Overall, my pants size has lowered from 52 to 40. My size 42 pants are now too big, and today I purchased two pair of size 40 pants. For dinner, I had my shake and an apple. I drank more water up until bedtime and had eight ounces before going to sleep.

Day 15

Today's weigh in was 256 lbs. I woke up this morning feeling well rest and energized. I drank 16 ounces of water with my medication when I got out of bed. Today was my second day in a row of doing my chi exercises. I'm still rusty. I did a set of the Perfect Push-up and bounced on my rebounder for 10 minutes. For breakfast, I had my shake and an apple. I went to my chiropractor to get a maintenance adjustment and then walked a mile and a half around the park. As I walked, I drank my water. My energy level was still high, so I decided to go to my martial arts class and got a great workout in. For lunch, I went to Chipotle (chicken, brown rice, peppers, black beans, salsa, and guacamole) since I was out and about. I was invited to two cookouts today and knew I would be surrounded by food I could not consume. I took my dinner (shake, almonds, and an apple) with me to the first cookout. At the second cookout, I just drank my water. I was somewhat surprised that I did not have the urge to eat at either event. When I returned home, I continued to drink water until bedtime and drank eight ounces before going to sleep.

Day 16

Today's weigh in was 256 lbs. This is my last week of cleansing. I woke up this morning feeling energized and drank 16 ounces of water with my medication upon getting out of bed. I did my chi, Perfect Push up, and rebounding exercises before I had my shake and apple for breakfast. I drank my water up until lunch. For lunch, I had a turkey burger with shrimp, brown rice, broccoli and raw carrots. My father and I are set to have dinner together for Father's Day. I will have my shake, apple, and almonds while he has the meal of his choosing. I continued to drink water up to having dinner with my father. At dinner, my father ordered several items that smelled so good, but I just had my shake and apple and enjoyed the great conversation we were having. After dinner, I continued to drink water up to bedtime and drank eight ounces before going to sleep.

Day 17

Today's weigh in was still 256 lbs. I woke up feeling pretty good and drank 16 ounces of water with my medication. I had to get to work earlier than normal, and since I didn't prepare my lunch the night before, I had to spend time this morning packing it. As a result of the lack of foresight, I didn't have time to do my morning exercises. For breakfast, I had my shake and apple. I had to sit in a training this morning and several of my colleagues chose to eat some chips. My mind fixated on the chips and the "urge to consume seed" was planted. I drank my water consistently up to lunch. For lunch, I had a turkey burger with shrimp, brown rice, broccoli, and raw carrots. The main difference today at lunch was while I was eating, I was still thinking about potato chips. I started drinking water again about an hour after lunch.

My water consumption was good throughout the day. For dinner, I had my shake and apple, but the chips were still on my mind. I began thinking, I could have some chips and no one would know. The beauty of journaling is that it helps with accountability and I did not want to write down that I caved in to the desire of having chips. In addition, my integrity won't let me lie to my readers. To help with this stronger than normal urge, I prayed to help remove the thoughts from my mind. I can honestly say I did not have those chips, even though I really wanted them. When I came home, I did my chi and Perfect Push-up exercises. I drank water for the rest of the evening and had eight ounces before going to sleep.

Day 18

Today's weigh in was 256 lbs. I have been holding steady at this weight for the past few days now. Since I have been doing the chi exercises, the tension in my neck, shoulders, and back have all subsided. I woke up feeling really good and had 16 ounces of water with my medicine upon getting out of bed. Yesterday, I purchased a new brand of protein powder for my shake and had it for breakfast. I prefer that taste to the other brand, but this one is more filling. I also dropped my vehicle off yesterday to be serviced and decided I would walk to the service shop from my house to pick it up. I somewhat underestimated the walking distance and travel time in getting to the shop and heading to work afterwards. I figured it would take me about 30 minutes to walk, and it turned out be about an hour to get to the shop. It turns out that the shop was 5 miles from my house. I didn't do my normal morning exercises, but the walk was a great substitute.

I drank my water consistently up to lunch. For lunch, it was the last of my turkey burger with shrimp, brown rice, broccoli, and raw carrots meals. I started drinking water again an hour later and continued drinking up to dinner. I packed my shake, an orange, and almonds with me for dinner, because I planned to go out to see a movie this evening. It is very important to plan for your success. I have made a few planning errors, and it did throw me off a bit. I have been consistent in preparing and eating my meals with the exception of Day 12. I had my shake and an orange for dinner while watching the movie. When I returned home, I did my chi and Perfect Push-up exercises. I drank water up until bedtime and drank eight ounces before going to sleep.

Day 19

Today's weigh in was still 256. Although the weight has not dropped over the past few days, I have noticed a change in my body composition. My clothes are fitting looser, and the contour of my body has definitely changed since beginning this cleansing. I woke up this morning before the alarm feeling energized. I had 16 ounces of water with my medication this morning, and my blood pressure read 117/69. I am really thrilled that my blood pressure is now under control and look forward to visiting my doctor in a few months to discuss ending the use of medication. Before having my shake for breakfast, I did my rebounding and Perfect Push-up exercises. I just realized that I neglected to mention that I start every morning off with a prayer of thankfulness for my life, health, and blessings. When I arrived at work, I was feeling quite energized, so I decided to run up the steps two at a time to the 5th floor. I made it without stopping.

I drank my water (56 ounces) consistently up to lunch. For lunch, I had salmon, quinoa, broccoli, and raw carrots. I began drinking water about an hour later. For a snack, I had raw almonds. I drank about 36 ounces of water up to dinner. Before I went home, I picked up my new bike and planned to ride it this evening to my martial arts class. For dinner, I had two small oranges and my shake. Since I knew I was going to have a pretty intense workout between riding the bike and going to class, I decided to eat two medium-sized bananas as well for some extra potassium. The workout I had—the bike ride (550 calories) and the activities of class—made those bananas come in handy. After I rode home, I did another set of the Perfect Push-up and my chi exercises. I drank water up to bedtime and had eight ounces before going to sleep.

Day 20

Today's weigh in was 254 lbs. Yesterday's activities really paid off. I woke up feeling energized yet again and had 16 ounces of water with my medication upon getting out of bed. I did a set of the Perfect Push-up before having my shake for breakfast. When I arrived at work, I ran the steps as I did yesterday to the 5th floor. That definitely had my blood flowing as I entered the presentation room. I just noticed that my water bottle actually holds 28 ounces and that I have been under reporting my water intake. Between waking up and lunch, I consumed 100 ounces of water. Based on my current body weight, I need to consume a minimum of 127 ounces daily. That is half my body weight. If you drink half your body weight in water throughout the day, you should see some positive results. For lunch, I had salmon, quinoa, broccoli, and raw carrots. I began drinking water again about an hour after lunch. For a snack, I had raw almonds. I drank 56 ounces of water up to dinner. For dinner, I had my shake and two bananas, because I am continuing my training for my upcoming martial arts tournament. When I returned home from my martial arts class, I only did my chi exercise, because my arms were sore from my martial arts workout. I drank eight ounces of water before going to sleep.

Day 21

Today's weigh in was 254 lbs. Today is the last day of cleansing, and I have lost 14 pounds over the 21 days. I woke up before the alarm today feeling full of energy. I drank 16 ounces of water with my medication upon getting out of bed. I decided to rest today and not do any exercise. For breakfast, I had my shake. I got off to a slow start in drinking my water while at work and only drank 20 ounces before lunch. For lunch, I had salmon, quinoa, broccoli, and raw carrots. My water intake increased after

52

lunch and I had 112 ounces before dinner. For dinner, I had my shake and two bananas. My energy level was good throughout the day. I drank water up to bedtime and had eight ounces before going to sleep.

I feel good about my accomplishment, because I was able to maintain the necessary commitment to achieve the results. There definitely were some moments where I felt like I would succumb to temptation, but I was able to press through. My energy level improved the further I got along in the cleansing. Within the past 21 days, I engaged in some intense activities and was able to make it through them without problems. I plan to continue to drink at least one shake a day for dinner about five days a week. My biggest challenge moving forward is not in the meals I eat, but how I will deal with those sudden urges to indulge in potato chips. There is nothing wrong with having chips occasionally. I just have a problem with over consumption when I choose to indulge. That is still something I must figure out. This second time of cleansing showed me like before that I don't need those seven types of food (eggs, dairy, corn, peanuts, sugar, gluten, and soy) to survive. I will reintroduce eggs, soy and corn to my diet periodically, but I see no real need to ever incorporate the rest.

Eight Steps to Take Before Attempting to Lose Weight

www.ingramcontent.com/pod-product-compliance
Lightning Source LLC
Chambersburg PA
CBHW070818290526
45795CB00002B/760